Dedicated to my mom, husband, grandparents, best friend Elizabeth, and all the wonderful members of Beautiful Purpose: A Bipolar Community Support Group and Nonprofit Organization.

The Bipolar Disorder Guide

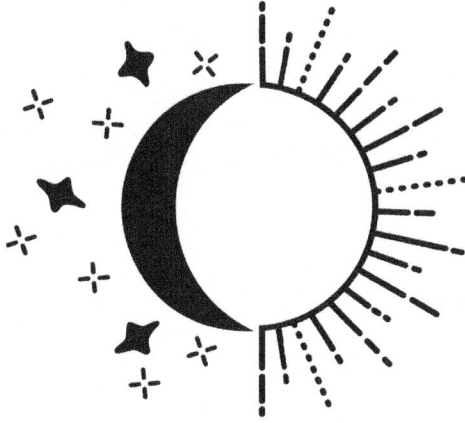

by Samantha Sunshine

Inspired by members of the

Support Group and Nonprofit Organization

Beautiful Purpose: A Bipolar Community

Join us on Facebook:

www.facebook.com/groups/BeautifulPurpose.BP

ISBN: 9798446646913

Independently published through Kindle Direct Publishing

Printed in the United States of America

Cover: Samantha Sunshine

Editing: Wendi Kelly

The use of this book implies your acceptance of these disclaimers:

This publication is sold with the understanding that the author and publisher are not engaged in rendering psychological, financial, legal, or other professional services. If expert assistance or counseling is needed, the services of a competent professional should be sought.

The advice herein is not intended to replace the services of trained health professionals, or be a substitute for medical advice. You are advised to consult with your health care professionals with regard to the matters relating to your health, and in particular with matters that may require diagnosis or medical attention, and the suggestions and recommendations made in this book.

The publisher and the author make no guarantees concerning the level of success you may experience by following the advice and strategies contained in this book, and you accept the risk that results will differ for each individual. The content of this book is for informational purposes only and is not intended to diagnose, treat, cure, or prevent any condition or disease.

Table of Contents

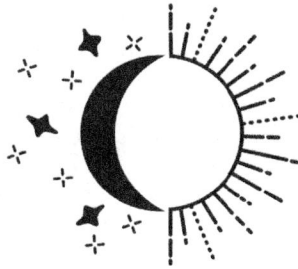

Do you or a loved one have Bipolar Disorder

and don't know where to start?

You are not alone.

So many members of Beautiful Purpose: A Bipolar Community describe the day they were diagnosed in the same way: They were told they have Bipolar Disorder, prescribed a new medication, and sent on their way with no information and no idea what to do next.

Inspired by the advice from members of Beautiful Purpose: A Bipolar Community, a support group and nonprofit organization, this short and simple guide includes everything we wish we'd known when we were first diagnosed.

There are so many great books out there that will tell you everything about Bipolar Disorder, but they can be overwhelming and hard to read. If you just want to know the basics of how to manage this illness and maintain stability, this is the place to start!

Join the Beautiful Purpose: A Bipolar Community group on Facebook:
www.facebook.com/groups/BeautifulPurpose.BP

About Samantha Sunshine and Beautiful Purpose: A Bipolar Community

My name is Samantha Sunshine, and I am a mental health advocate, founder of Beautiful Purpose: A Bipolar Community nonprofit organization and Facebook support group, and now, to my delight, an author. There was a time when I never would have imagined being any of these things. It was by wholeheartedly claiming my disorder and making a commitment to managing it, that this came to be.

I was diagnosed with Bipolar Disorder in late 2015, and was quite lost for many years. I kept my diagnosis a secret and went blindly through the obstacles of this illness. The struggles I went through and the darkness I faced were unbearable at times, and I honestly thought I was the only one going through the experience.

In 2019, I was depressed and alone, when it came to my mind that there may be some support groups on Facebook for people with Bipolar Disorder. Sure enough I found plenty, and I began to cry happy tears when I found them. "I found my people!" I told my husband. The experience of finding out I wasn't the only one going through these struggles was life-changing.

While I was incredibly grateful for these support groups, I craved a more positive and encouraging place to find comfort and support. I decided to make my own group for people with Bipolar Disorder, with the plan of posting motivational quotes and inspiring people to share positive experiences they had instead of just their struggles.

This group gave me the freedom to express myself and talk openly about my journey, while encouraging others to push through and find happiness. The group grew, and grew, and I was in awe as it remained a positive, uplifting place to be. People not only asked for support but shared everything about their journey, including the positives. It was more than a support group, it was a "community". We got to know each other's stories and there was always positive encouragement in the comments and posts.

After a year of running the group, I gained enough confidence and comfort in myself that I announced to everyone I knew that I had Bipolar Disorder. I was (and still am) proud to be living my life to the fullest despite my challenges. I was no longer depressed, but I continued to be active in the group because it uplifted me to help others who were going through what I went through alone. I didn't want anyone to feel the way I did for so many years. I also wanted all of us to be able to gain a greater understanding of Bipolar Disorder, so I put together a book club where we could read and learn about it together. I started a fundraiser to provide books to members, and it was so successful that I realized I truly had the ability to make a difference in people's lives.

Around the same time, I happened to meet someone who had founded a nonprofit organization. I was immediately inspired to do the same. I began researching how to make a nonprofit organization and blindly navigated my way through the endless paperwork it took to create it. I received amazing support from the group.

This opened up so many opportunities. I started thinking about what else I could do to help people. Pill organizers came to mind. My pill organizer is a life-saver and one of the main factors in maintaining my stability, so I started a fundraiser and provided them to members. The possibilities were endless from there. We now provide books about Bipolar Disorder, pill organizers, journals, planners, weighted blankets, coping items, self care items, and many other tools for living with this disorder and maintaining stability.

My next goal is to help those with Bipolar Disorder by guiding them through the process of reaching and maintaining stability. I have been asking the members of Beautiful Purpose: A Bipolar Community what they wish they had known when they were first diagnosed, and compiled this book with all of their feedback (as well as my own). I've combed through every detail to make sure I don't leave anything out, with the hopes that you will start out with the great advantage of knowing what to do along the way. Thank you for picking up this guide. I hope it helps you on your journey!

~Samantha Sunshine

Diagnosis

"It was really freeing to have the information [of being diagnosed with bipolar disorder]. It made me really happy because I started to have a relationship with myself, and I think that's the best part. Like, I've probably been the happiest I've ever been."
~Selena Gomez (Singer, actress, producer, and entrepreneur)

Everyone responds to their Bipolar Disorder diagnosis differently. You may be upset, scared, confused, indifferent, or even relieved. Any response you have is valid, and you have a right to go through the different emotions it may bring. Through education, research, reflection, and connecting with others who also have Bipolar Disorder, you can reach an acceptance and understanding of your diagnosis.

Try to go through this process with an open mind, knowing your initial response can change over time. The "unknown" is scary and intimidating, so you may feel better once you learn more about it. Although it might not be your first reaction, it's important to come to an acceptance of your diagnosis so you can take the next step toward living a stable life.

A diagnosis is just an explanation of what you've experienced and an indicator of what kind of medication, therapy, and treatment you need. Being diagnosed correctly can be a very positive thing, as it is the beginning of your journey to stability and fulfillment. With this new diagnosis, you can finally discover the right plan to overcome the challenges of the disorder you've been facing all along.

What is Bipolar Disorder?

Bipolar Disorder, previously called Manic Depression, is a mental illness known for causing significant changes in a person's mood, energy, and ability to function. These changes, or "episodes," can last days, weeks, months, or even years. It would be impossible to get into the scientific reasoning behind Bipolar Disorder in such a short guide, but what's most important for you to know is that it's not something you've caused or learned. It's an illness scientifically caused by chemical imbalances, complications in the way your brain functions, and the genes you carry. It's a biological disorder that you had no part in causing.

Types of Bipolar Disorder

There are different types of Bipolar Disorder depending on what kinds of mood episodes you experience. At this point in your diagnosis, you might not know which type of Bipolar Disorder you have. That's okay! What's important is that you know you have Bipolar Disorder in general. This means you can begin treatment and learn how to manage and cope with your illness.

The most common forms of Bipolar Disorder and the types of episodes they experience are:

- **Bipolar type 1:** Mania, Hypomania, and Depression.

- **Bipolar type 2:** Hypomania and Depression. (No Mania)

- **Cyclothymia:** Mood episodes that are more mild than hypomania or depression, but significant enough to warrant a diagnosis.

Types of Mood Episodes

Mania: Mania is a period of feeling extremely high energy lasting at least one week, or less if hospitalization is necessary.

Mania may include the following symptoms:

- Increase in energy or psychomotor agitation (restlessness, inability to sit still, purposeless movements such as pacing, etc.)
- Decreased need for sleep
- More talkative than usual or feeling pressure to keep talking
- Racing thoughts or flight of ideas
- Distractibility
- Inflated self-esteem or thoughts of grandeur
- Taking part in pleasurable activities that may have negative consequences, such as (but not limited to):
  - Spending more money than usual
  - Gambling
  - Making risky and/or unusual investments
  - Driving recklessly and/or speeding
  - Having risky sexual encounters or experiencing hypersexuality
  - Using drugs and/or alcohol
- Sometimes mania includes psychotic symptoms, such as:
  - Visual (sight), auditory (sound), tactile (touch), gustatory (taste), and/or olfactory (smell) hallucinations.
  - Delusions, or believing in things that are not real, such as thinking you can read people's minds, believing you are God, being convinced that you're going to be famous, thinking you're being tracked or that people are out to get you, and/or having other bizarre or untrue beliefs.

Types of Mania

- **Euphoric Mania:** In euphoric mania, the excess energy comes in the form of elation, happiness, excitement, and/or a type of exhilaration. One may enjoy risk-taking and thrilling activities such as gambling, spending more money than usual, coming up with grand ideas, having high confidence in themselves, drinking more alcohol than usual, experimenting with or becoming addicted to drugs, making risky sexual decisions, and more. Often, people experiencing mania don't realize the effects of the decisions they are making. It is not until they fall into a depression or become stable that they realize the wake of destruction left in their path. Psychosis is not a required symptom, but if it does occur it can involve being overly religious or spiritual, believing they can read thoughts and/or communicate telepathically, see "signs" and synchronicities, and more. Overall, this can feel like a good experience but have destructive consequences.

- **Dysphoric Mania:** Dysphoric mania, also called "mixed mania" or a "mixed episode", includes excess energy accompanied by feelings of being depressed, overwhelmed, irritable, angry, and/or other negative emotions. One may find themselves making risky and dangerous decisions such as driving recklessly, spending more money than usual, drinking more alcohol than usual, experimenting with or becoming addicted to drugs, and more. Psychosis sometimes accompanied with dysphoric mania is often scary and unpleasant. "Shadow people" are a common hallucination reported by people experiencing dysphoric mania. These are shadows seen out of the corner of the eye that can be frightening. It can also involve paranoia, voices, believing people are watching or listening, and other disturbing beliefs. Overall, this can feel like a very bad experience and result in destructive consequences.

Hypomania: Hypomania is an episode of high energy that is not severe enough to warrant hospitalization or debilitate the person from working or doing regular activities. All the symptoms of mania apply (except psychosis), but in a milder form. Hypomania lasts at least 4 days.

Hypomania may include the following symptoms:

- Increase in energy or psychomotor agitation (restlessness, inability to sit still, purposeless movements such as pacing, etc.)

- Decreased need for sleep
- More talkative than usual or feeling pressure to keep talking
- Racing thoughts or flight of ideas
- Distractibility
- Inflated self-esteem or thoughts of grandeur
- Taking part in pleasurable activities that may have negative consequences, such as (but not limited to):
    - Spending more money than usual
    - Gambling
    - Making risky and/or unusual investments
    - Driving recklessly and/or speeding
    - Having risky sexual encounters or experiencing hypersexuality
    - Using drugs and/or alcohol
- No psychotic symptoms.

Euthymia: Euthymia is a fancy way of saying "stability." We are not always manic, hypomanic, or depressed. We go through periods of stable moods as well.

Depression: Depressive episodes can be mild, moderate, or severe depending on the impact on regular activities and work functioning. A major depressive episode is characterized by a severely depressed mood lasting at least two weeks.

Depression may include the following symptoms:

- Depressed mood
- Loss of interest or pleasure in activities
- Significant weight gain or loss
- Decrease or increase in appetite
- Moving and/or talking slower than usual
- Engaging in purposeless movements such as pacing, etc.
- Fatigue or loss of energy
- Feelings of worthlessness or guilt
- Diminished ability to think or concentrate, and/or indecisiveness
- Recurrent thoughts of death, suicidal ideation, or a suicide attempt

Mixed Episodes: A mixed episode, also called "dysphoric mania" or "mixed mania" (as mentioned on page 13), is when major symptoms of two different types of episodes are present at the same time. This means there are three or more symptoms of mania present, while there are also three or more symptoms of depression present. One example would be if they were majorly depressed but have high energy, racing thoughts, and are making risky decisions. See page 12 "Mania" and page 15 "Depression" for possible symptoms of a mixed episode.

What Should I Do Now?

"There is no need to suffer silently and there is no shame in seeking help."
~Catherine Zeta-Jones (Actress)

Now that you've learned a bit about what your diagnosis is, you might be wondering what to do about it. That's where this guide comes in handy. Members of the Beautiful Purpose: A Bipolar Community group have shared all the things they wish they had known when they were first diagnosed, and it all begins right after diagnosis.

Here are the first things you should do now that you are diagnosed.

- **Find a good psychiatrist** who listens to your symptoms and side effects and makes the medication adjustments as needed. Remember that a psychiatrist has years of education in treating mental illnesses, so their suggestions and the adjustments they recommend are important to follow.

- **Find a therapist that works with you**. According to members of the Beautiful Purpose: A Bipolar Community group, therapy is one of the most important parts of managing and coping with Bipolar Disorder. A good therapist will listen to all of your thoughts without judgment and offer insightful advice on how to move forward in healthy ways. (See page 20 "Therapy" for details).

- **Make a promise to yourself** that you will stay on top of scheduling and attending all appointments. It's easy to fall behind, but remember it is the most important thing you need to do in order to reach and maintain stability. Also, if you don't go to your psychiatrist often enough they sometimes will not refill your prescriptions.

- **Take your medication as prescribed**. (See page 18 "Medication" for tips). Note: *never* stop your medication without the help of your psychiatrist. This can cause physical and mental reactions sending you to the hospital or inpatient psychiatric care.

- **Educate yourself**. Reading this guide to learn things you need to know to find stability and successfully manage your illness is a great start. We've included everything we wish we had known when we were first diagnosed so we can help *you*. While many of the topics may seem irrelevant to you now, they will be extremely useful to you on this journey towards stability and a fulfilling life. Keep this guide handy so you can refer back to it at any time.

- **Post in the Beautiful Purpose: A Bipolar Community group** whenever you need encouragement, have questions, or simply need to talk about what you're going through. We are a very welcoming and supportive community!

Medication

"There is treatment and a variety of medications that can alleviate your symptoms if you are manic depressive or depressive."

~Carrie Fisher (Writer and actress, known for her role as

Princess Leia in Star Wars)

Medication is a key factor in finding and maintaining stability. Remember that the brain is an organ in the body. Just like a diabetic needs insulin to help the pancreas balance blood sugar levels, we need medication to balance the chemicals in our brain. Medication is nothing to be ashamed of. In fact, it is a miracle. We have to be honest here: It's not always easy finding the right medication. However, with patience and perseverance you can reach stability and fulfillment.

Here are some things you need to know:

- **Be prepared to experiment.** Finding the right medication is a trial-and-error process. Along the way some may make you feel better and some may make you feel worse. It's *so* important and *so* worth it to stick through this process! Remember you are investing in the rest of your life.

- **Always communicate** all symptoms and side effects with your psychiatrist so the right adjustments can be made.

- **Be your own advocate!** Unfortunately sometimes our concerns are dismissed by doctors, and it's important that we are persistent until they are addressed. If something isn't working, speak up, and keep speaking until you are heard.

- **Be patient!** Medications take 3-8 weeks to start working. Ask your doctor to find out how long it should take a specific medication to become effective.

- **Treatment almost always takes more than one medication.** It will usually include an antidepressant to prevent you from becoming depressed and a mood stabilizer to prevent you from having any other mood episodes. Antipsychotics are also commonly prescribed and have a variety of purposes: They can help improve your mood and prevent mania and/or psychosis, among other things.

- **Take your pills at the same time every day.** Use an alarm to help remind you. This will ensure your medication is most effective. Note: *never* stop medication without speaking to your doctor. This can cause physical and mental reactions sending you to the hospital or inpatient psychiatric care.

- **Use a Pill Organizer.** A pill organizer truly makes taking medication much more simple and convenient. It will help you make sure you don't forget your pills or take them twice by accident. It also allows you to see when you need refills ahead of time so you don't accidentally run out. This is extremely important if you want to be stable.

Therapy

"Therapy is not to 'talk about' things, but to change the person's life, and to relieve suffering, such as depression, anxiety, or relationship problems."

~David D. Burns, MD (Psychiatrist and author)

"It's incredibly liberating to spend an hour talking to someone and not caring about what you sound like. It's about understanding myself."

~Shakira (Singer)

Countless members of the Beautiful Purpose: A Bipolar Community group testify that therapy is one of the other key factors in finding and maintaining stability. One thing people who have never been to therapy often say is, "Why would I pay someone to talk to me?" The truth is that it's far from just talking to someone about your feelings. Therapy is invaluable. You'll just have to trust us on this one.

Here is some guidance we've put together to help you commit to therapy:

- **Find a therapist that works for you.** Not just any therapist, but one who truly is compatible with you. This may take trying more than one to find someone you are comfortable with. Never be afraid to switch to a new therapist; This is a normal part of the process. Keep trying until you feel heard and validated.

- **Know that therapy takes time**. It can be difficult or awkward at first. It takes awhile to develop a comfortable and open relationship with your therapist. You will get the most out of therapy if you are vulnerable and honest with them, so allowing yourself to be truthful about your deepest feelings is important.

- **Therapists can be valuable wealths of information**. Therapists can share tools and provide resources you likely won't find on your own. They can find the type of therapy that is right for you, teach you coping skills in detail that will help you greatly (see brief examples on page 25 "Coping Skills"), as well as connect you with groups and programs that may be beneficial to you.

- **Therapists can help you process any past traumas.** You will feel so much better once you've overcome the deep-rooted issues that have been holding you back. You deserve to feel free from any past negative experiences you've had!

- **Therapists are there for *you*** during all points of your life in any way you need them to be. They're not just there to be someone to talk to, they can also help you set goals and hold you accountable for any accomplishments you'd like to make. These can vary from reaching long-term life goals, to healing from trauma, to helping with self care, and anything else you can think of.

- **Therapy Time is Your Time.** Remember your therapist went into this field because they want to help people. You are never wasting their time by venting your grievances and sharing your stories. They are there for *you,* and believe it or not they actually want to listen and help!

Lifestyle

"Bipolar in some regards has been a blessing because it's been a catalyst to make the changes in my life that I needed to make. That manic episode shattered me, it was an immense embarrassment, humiliation — but had that not happened I wouldn't be where I am today, rebuilding my life, my career, a more stable 'me' that I haven't been in 20 years."
~Scott Stapp, former Creed frontman

Successfully managing Bipolar Disorder means having a structured lifestyle and changing many habits and activities you may be used to. This can be a very positive thing, as it provides the opportunity to live a healthier, more well-rounded life! While it may take some work to get used to your new habits and routines, it is absolutely worth it. Embrace this new lifestyle as a chance to start fresh on your journey to fulfillment.

Here are some of the main things you will want to focus on to achieve and maintain stability:

- **Sleep**: It is extremely important to maintain a consistent sleep schedule. Sleep disturbances are known to be one of the causes of episodes. Getting too little or too much sleep can cause mania, hypomania, or depression. When you are manic or hypomanic, it is especially important to get enough sleep. If you're having trouble sleeping, talk to your psychiatrist. You may need to be prescribed a medication to help fall asleep and stay asleep.

- **Self Care**: Keeping up with self care is one of the most important parts of managing and coping with this disorder. When we practice self care, we keep ourselves in a consistent routine and improve our overall wellness. (See page 24 "Self Care" for more information).

- **Stay sober**: Yes, it's true, we need to stay away from all drugs and alcohol. They can cause interactions with our medication, causing decreased or increased efficacy, resulting in seizures, blackouts, and more. Drugs and alcohol can also cause episodes. Many members of the Beautiful Purpose: A Bipolar Community group say one of the best things they did to manage their disorder was cut out drugs and alcohol completely.

- **Routine:** It's important to keep a routine. Go to sleep and wake up at the same time every day as much as possible. Create a routine for self care, such as taking time to relax and restore your energy each day, showering on certain days of the week, and brushing your hair and teeth daily.

- **Exercise:** A healthy body nurtures a healthy mind. There are countless activities to get your body moving and to be active. Some ideas to get you started are: Walking, running, hiking, yoga, aerobics, swimming, sports, cycling, strength training, pilates, dancing, martial arts, kickboxing, etc.

Self Care

"It's possible to live well, feel well, and also find happiness with Bipolar Disorder or any other mental illness [you're] struggling with."
~ Demi Lovato (Singer, songwriter, and actress)

People with Bipolar Disorder can become overstimulated or exhausted by events, people, activities, work, and more. It's important to rest and recharge after expending any mental or physical energy in order to maintain stability and overall wellness.

Here are some of the ways you can take care of yourself:

- **Always keep up with the basics**: Eat food, drink water, sleep, and take showers (once every 3 days at the least). Sometimes when we are hypomanic or manic, we can forget to cover the basics, and in depression we can feel too exhausted to do anything. In times of difficulty, be sure to make yourself accomplish the basics.

- **Self care favorites**. Make a list of self care activities you can refer to for restoring your body, mind, and soul. Having this list handy will help in times when you are unable to come up with something on your own. You can find an infinite number of self care ideas on the internet. Some ideas from the Beautiful Purpose: A Bipolar Community group are: Soak in a hot bath, take a refreshing shower, go on a walk, spend time in nature, read a book, listen to music, journal, cook, bake, paint your nails, color in a coloring book, create art, exercise, do yoga, stretch, use essential oils, light a candle, garden, etc.

- **Spend time in nature**. Being in nature is a form of self care. It is refreshing, rejuvenating, and a great way to "escape" our lives for a while. Whether it's sitting outside in the fresh air or going on hikes, it can be great for your body and mind.

- **Don't feel like you're alone.** Feel free to ask for encouragement and share your self care activities in the Beautiful Purpose: A Bipolar Community group! We love to see what each other are doing to relax, rejuvenate, and take care of ourselves!

Coping Skills

"At times, being Bipolar can be an all-consuming challenge, requiring a lot of stamina and even more courage, so if you're living with this illness and functioning at all, it's something to be proud of, not ashamed of."

~Carrie Fisher (Writer and actress)

Since Bipolar Disorder is known for causing significant changes in our moods, energy, and functioning, it's essential to learn coping skills so we can continue our everyday tasks and responsibilities during difficult times.

Here are some tips to help build coping skills.

- **Make a Plan for Fun**. Remember to do things that make you happy. While you are doing well, make a list of enjoyable activities that you can refer to at any time. Just like having a list of self care activities is beneficial, having a list of ways to remove ourselves from overwhelming situations is important, too.

- **Journaling is one of the most important coping skills to practice.** This is highly recommended by therapists and members of the Beautiful Purpose: A Bipolar Community group. (See page 32 "Use a Journal or Notebook").

- **Exercise is a great coping mechanism**. A healthy body is important for a healthy mind, and even just the psychological effects of exercise can have a positive effect on your life. Exercise helps expel excess energy, irritability, anger, and any other intense emotions you experience.

- **Yoga is amazing for your body, mind, and soul.** Just doing five minutes of yoga can help reset your thoughts and stretch your body so it feels good. Look up "Beginning Yoga Routine" on YouTube and you will find plenty of guidance if you've never done it. You can do this to start your day, release tension in your body and mind, or to wind down at the end of the day.

- **Meditation is a highly recommended coping skill.** To give your mind a break from your anxious or busy thoughts, meditation is very beneficial to your overall well-being. Remember that it's okay not to be good at it at first. It takes practice and is very rewarding once you get the hang of it. Youtube and apps like Calm and Headspace are great for help learning how to meditate.

- **Pets are very helpful for coping!** Depending on what type of pet you have, you can cuddle with them, play with them, or take them on walks. They also give you purpose and a reason to get out of bed on bad days. You can talk to your psychiatrist to make your pet an official Emotional Support Animal.

- **Practice Mindfulness.** Mindfulness is a very helpful tool for coping with Bipolar Disorder. Therapists often teach mindfulness, but there are also many videos, books, and workbooks that you can use to learn how to practice it as well. Mindfulness focuses on being in the present moment instead of worrying about the past or future, and accepting your feelings, thoughts, and emotions as they come and go. Accepting what you are experiencing helps remove any resistance that could be holding you back from finding peace in the present moment.

- **Listening to music is a great way to release energy or shift your mood.** Music can truly affect our moods and heal our soul. Choose any type of music to either release the tension you are holding or to shift your energy to a more positive emotion. Listening to music you relate to while in a certain mood and connecting to the sounds and/or lyrics is a great way to start. Then, transition to a soothing genre to shift into a more relaxed state. Some soothing genres include classical, slow jazz, chillstep, or choir music.

- **Discover the importance of self-compassion.** Sometimes when we're not performing as well as we'd like to be, we turn to self-blame and disappointment. We need to give ourselves grace. Books and workbooks can help guide you through the process of discovering self-compassion.

Grounding Techniques

"Grounding" is a method that can be used at any time, especially during anxiety attacks or before and after stressful events. There are an infinite number of grounding techniques. You can find these on the internet, in the Beautiful Purpose: A Bipolar Community group, or by talking to your therapist.

Here are some examples of grounding techniques:

- **Relax**. One of the easiest ways to ground yourself is to unclench your jaw, drop your shoulders, take a deep breath, and feel the tension release from your body. You can do this discreetly at any time during the day.

- **The 5 4 3 2 1 technique** helps you focus on your five senses instead of anxious or triggering thoughts. It's quite easy: when feeling overwhelmed, name 5 things you can see, 4 things you can hear, 3 things you can touch, 2 things you can smell, and 1 thing you can taste. You'd be surprised by how effective this is, especially during panic attacks!

- **Focus on your breathing**. Forms of meditation that concentrate on the breath are very beneficial for grounding. Different breathing rhythms can promote relaxation, awareness, distress tolerance, energy levels, focus, and tension release. This is called Paced Breathing. Simply repeat the breathing patterns below for different effects:

  - Extended Exhale: Inhale 4 seconds - Exhale 6 seconds.

  - Balance Breathing: Inhale 4 seconds - Exhale 2 seconds.

  - Restorative: Inhale 5 seconds - Exhale 5 seconds.

  - Focus: Inhale 4 seconds - Exhale 4 seconds.

  - Energize: Inhale 4 seconds - Exhale 2 seconds.

  - Relaxation: Inhale 4 seconds - Exhale 7 seconds - Inhale 8 seconds - Exhale 8 seconds.

- **The T.I.P.S. Method** works by changing body chemistry to help gain better control over intense emotions and reactions to triggering events.

  - Temperature: Placing cold water or an icepack across the eyes and forehead helps regulate your body's reaction to extreme emotions.

  - Physical exercise: Vigorous activity helps expend built up energy to allow you to gain control over intense emotional reactions.

  - Paired Muscle Relaxation: Systematic tensing and relaxing of muscle groups helps you calm and ground yourself. (You can find instructions online or look up videos on YouTube).

  - Self-soothing: Engaging the five senses with soothing and pleasurable experiences is a great coping and grounding tool during times of emotional distress. Some examples you can use are soothing lights, soft music, sour candy (yes this helps!), essential oils, and cozy blankets.

- **Taking a mindful walk** can relax your mind and bring you to the present moment. A "mindful walk", which is also known as a walking meditation, is when you take in your surroundings, observing one thing at a time and paying close attention to your senses: Noticing the shape of clouds, the individual leaves in the trees, or the birds flying through the sky. Or, it could be listening to the sounds of your steps, chirping of the birds, or paying attention to the feeling of the warmth of the sun or coolness of a breeze on your skin. Inhaling the smell of the freshly cut lawn or someone's dinner being made and noticing your reactions are all examples of mindful walking.

- **Practicing self care and coping activities** can be used as grounding techniques. Using the lists you created in the "Self Care" section on page 24 and the "Coping Skills" section on page 25, choose something you can easily do when you're in a time of distress. Perhaps a nice hot bath or listening to music would help bring you peace of mind and feel grounded.

If You Notice Signs of an Episode

"Time will pass; these moods will pass; and I will, eventually, be myself again."

~ Kay Redfield Jamison PhD, MA (Former Professor of Psychiatry and author of

An Unquiet Mind: A Memoir of Moods and Madness)

If you notice signs of an episode, it's important to immediately take action. The sooner you take action, the less of an impact the episode will have on you. The first thing to do is make an appointment with your psychiatrist and therapist. You may need a medication adjustment to get you back on track.

Here are some instructions on what else to do during the different episodes:

Hypomania or Mania:

- **Try to slow down by using coping and grounding techniques.** (Pages 25-28).

- **Limit activities.** Often when we are hypomanic or manic we want and feel capable of doing many activities and want to make many plans. While this may be tempting, do not fall for it. Activities, people, and events can easily wear us out. Although we may feel like we can do anything, we need to maintain caution and understand that these things do catch up to us. The difference is instead of affecting us that same day or following day, they will affect us when we "come down" from the episode.

- **Do not make long-term commitments.** While it's natural to want to start projects and have new ideas when hypomanic or manic, we sometimes cannot follow through once the episode is over. Write down your new ideas, and wait until you are stable to make any promises or commitments.

- **Pay attention to your spending.** Hypomania and mania can make you want to spend money, and this can cause negative consequences. Some ideas for limiting spending include leaving your debit card at home and only using cash, and removing your card number from all online shopping websites.

- **Do NOT use drugs or alcohol.** This can be very dangerous and lead to disastrous and long-term negative consequences.

Depression:

- **Practice self care, no matter how hard it is.** It's easy to let self care fall to the wayside while we are having a hard time doing anything, but keeping up with our hygiene is very important. The more we "let ourselves go", the deeper we will fall into depression. There are many apps to help you keep track of your self care. Finch is a free app often recommended by members of the Beautiful Purpose: A Bipolar Community group.

- **Keep a routine.** This truly helps! While it's tempting to stay in bed all day, keeping a routine will help keep you from falling into a deeper depression.

- **Stay active, even if it's just a little bit.** Going on a short walk, even if it's just down the street, can be very beneficial. The fresh air and sunlight can bring positive effects to your mood and overall health. Doing a short yoga routine or even just some stretches can help you get your blood flowing and be more able to do self care and keep your routine.

- **Share your achievements in the Beautiful Purpose: A Bipolar Community group!** When everything is hard, we recognize that it is a huge accomplishment to take and celebrate small steps and we will be there to support and congratulate you for all the little things, like taking a shower or eating.

- **Contact a crisis line if you're having any thoughts of suicide:**
  - Call or text 988 for the Suicide & Crisis Linfeline
  - Go to www.988Lifeline.org to chat with someone online
  - Call 911 if you have a plan for suicide, or are a threat to yourself or others

Have a Crisis Plan

During your journey, you may at some point need to be admitted to inpatient care. You may be incapacitated due to severe depression, mania, or psychosis, among other factors. In case this ever happens, it's important to have a plan prepared ahead of time.

Some ideas of what your crisis plan should include:

- ☐ Your preferred facility you would like to be admitted to

- ☐ Names, addresses, phone numbers, and emails of your healthcare team

    - ☐ Primary care physician

    - ☐ Psychiatrist

    - ☐ Therapist

- ☐ Your insurance information

- ☐ List of medications and allergies

- ☐ Phone numbers of loved ones and/or friends

- ☐ A checklist so you don't forget anything you want to bring:

    - ☐ Clothing with no strings, straps, or zippers

    - ☐ A journal or notebook

    - ☐ Books to read

    - ☐ Stress toy for anxiety, such as fidget items

    - ☐ Flip flops for showering

    - ☐ Toothpaste and toothbrush

    - ☐ Shampoo and conditioner

    - ☐ Favorite lotion or essential oils

Use a Journal or Notebook

A journal or notebook is a necessity for you throughout this journey. There are many uses for it besides writing down your thoughts (although that is helpful in itself). Having a place to document everything you experience will be very beneficial and a great way to review your progress, patterns, and daily reflections.

In your journal or notebook you can:

- **Document your week**. Many of us find that when we go to the psychiatrist or therapist we forget what we wanted to talk about. Use your journal or notebook to write down things that happen during the week, and/or things you'd like to bring up at your appointment. You can make bullet points or write full sentences and paragraphs to read out loud. It may sound strange to recite something at your appointment, but it's extremely useful and makes things a lot easier!

- **Track your moods!** Tracking your moods in a journal or notebook can help you, your psychiatrist, and your therapist identify what you're going through and how to help. You can do this by rating your mood on a number scale each day, or by creating a chart to help you visualize your moods. Note: Apps such as Daylio are extremely helpful and easy to use for mood tracking as well. There is a small subscription fee for Daylio, but it is worth paying for your mental health. At the time this guide is being written it is $2.99/mo.

- **Reflection and patterns**. Writing in a journal and going back to reflect can help you identify your triggers, symptoms, and signs of episodes. This will prove to be very useful during your journey for you, your therapist, and your psychiatrist.

- **Medication changes and symptoms**. Paying close attention during medication changes is extremely important. Write down any symptoms and/or side effects while trying new medications or making adjustments. Take it with you to your psychiatrist appointment. Do not discard these as they could be handy well into the future if a medication change is ever needed.

- **Emptying your mind**. Get out your thoughts, stories, poetry, doodles, and anything else you can think of in a journal or notebook. It's very therapeutic to put these out of your mind and onto a paper, especially if you are ruminating (repeating the same thoughts over and over again), anxious, or excited about something.

The Importance of Art and Creativity

"Writing is a form of therapy; sometimes I wonder how all those who do not write, compose or paint can manage to escape the madness, melancholia, the panic and fear which is inherent in a human situation."

~Graham Greene (Author and journalist)

"I try to take what's going on and turn it into something beautiful in the best way that I can."

~Selena Gomez (Singer, actress, producer, and entrepreneur)

Being creative is a very therapeutic coping skill. It can remove you from your current circumstances and give you the opportunity to channel your feelings into something tangible that you can reflect on and process in a new, healthier way.

- **Embrace a broad definition of art** and embark on a creative journey. You don't need to be good to create something! Remember, it's about the experience, not the destination. Have no expectations of what the outcome will be. Just go for it!

- **Channel your emotions into a masterpiece.** You might surprise yourself with what your hands and mind can create when going through intense emotions. Creating your own masterpiece brings a sense of accomplishment and pride. It's a wonderful thing to transform intense feelings into something beautiful.

- **You can make art through any medium:** Paint, markers, pens, old recycled materials, colored pencils, stickers, pictures, fabric, yarn, and anything else you can possibly think of. Challenge yourself to use any medium to create something personal. Remember that being abstract is a type of art, too!

- **Words are also art**. You can be creative through visual art as well as good old pen and paper. Poetry, lyrics, stories, novels, and memoirs are all ways to be creative with words.

- **Where to begin:** If you're stumped on where to start, Google "Art Therapy Prompts". You will find many wonderful prompts to get you started on your creative journey.

- **Share your work** in the Beautiful Purpose: A Bipolar Community group! Artwork is something that makes the group a "community" instead of just a support group. We love to see what others are creating and give our interpretations of what the work is expressing (if the creator wants us to).

Finding Acceptance and Forgiveness

Everyone responds to their new diagnosis differently. If you feel any resistance to your diagnosis, remember this: With this new diagnosis you can get the right medication, therapy, and overall treatment you need. Although this may not be your initial thought or reaction, it's important to start to view it this way so you can make progress towards stability.

- **Focus on the positive**. In coming to terms with the diagnosis and how you see yourself, nurture a positive mindset. Welcome the new perspective on your life as a step towards understanding who you are and ways you can live a fulfilling life.

- **Getting Answers**. After you're diagnosed, you can finally understand the reason for the feelings and experiences you've had in the past. Many say they thought they had caused whatever was wrong with them. This brought guilt, anger, shame, and self-loathing. This diagnosis proves they were simply coping with something that was beyond their control at the time. There was a biological reason for what they were going through. For this reason, we can forgive ourselves and understand that our experiences were valid.

- **Let go of guilt**. In looking back at decisions you made before beginning treatment, realize that you didn't have all the information you needed to choose the best path. Your judgment was impaired due to biological reasons. Let go of any guilt you may have surrounding that time in your life. You cannot go back and change them, so you must forgive yourself, learn from them, and make amends wherever possible.

- **Find comfort in acceptance**. Forgiveness is rooted in acceptance. If you can't imagine forgiving yourself or someone else, focus on accepting what happened and finding comfort in having the opportunity to move forward.

Opening Up to Others

"I am mentally ill. I can say that. I am not ashamed of that. I survived that, I'm still surviving it, but bring it on."
~Carrie Fisher (Author and actress)

Opening up to others can be scary because we have no way of knowing how they will react. Unfortunately, there is a stigma around mental health, most likely stemming from the fact that many people don't know a lot about mental illnesses or the importance of mental health in general. When opening up to others, it's important to be ready with facts and information to clarify any misconceptions or misinformation they have. Oftentimes, education brings understanding.

Here are some tips to help you open up to others:

- **Educate yourself** and be ready to answer any questions they might have.

- **Write down what you'd like to say beforehand**. This will help you make sure you don't forget something you want to say or get nervous on the spot and say things differently than you had planned.

- **Start by telling one person you trust**. Be open, honest, and ready for whatever reaction they may have.

- **Have patience** while they process this information. It can be unexpected and come as a shock to them. If their first reaction is not ideal, keep in mind it may evolve into acceptance, support, and understanding over time.

- **Their reaction doesn't define you.** Remember that no matter what someone else thinks, it doesn't change who you are, the hard work you are putting in, and what you are learning about yourself. You're asking for support and understanding. The right people will see this and appreciate you for who you are.

- **Brains are a part of the body too**. One idea that you might find comfort in sharing is that people with mental illness are not that different from people who have chronic physical illnesses. Bipolar Disorder is a chronic illness of the brain. For example, people with diabetes have to take insulin to make up for what their pancreas doesn't produce, while we have to take medication to balance the chemicals that our brain produces. Both the pancreas and the brain are organs in our body that for some people need help functioning!

What Can Others Do to Help?

Having an understanding supportive person can be very helpful in managing this disorder. They are able to pick up on things we might not notice, such as signs that an episode is coming or that we've forgotten to take our medication. However, it takes good communication, honesty and some introspection to teach them how best to support us.

Here are some things others can do to help, and ways we can *help* them help us:

- **Learn your signs, symptoms, and triggers.** Oftentimes others are able to recognize these before we can, and that can help prevent full episodes. By being aware of these things, and sharing them with our support team, we can take the necessary steps to prevent a severe episode from occurring.

- **Learn to accept help graciously**. Accepting help from others when they point out our signs and symptoms is very important. They can be a valuable asset for maintaining stability. If you find yourself getting defensive, talk to them about how you would like them to approach the topic in a way that will make you feel better in the future. Communication throughout this journey is extremely important.

- **Educate themselves.** Those who want to support you can watch YouTube videos, find articles, read books, and ask questions. (See pages 40-41 for "Informational / Help Books", "Memoirs", "Podcasts", and "Websites"). Sometimes it helps to research the scientific explanation for Bipolar Disorder.

- **Fill up your pill organizer each week.** This can be extremely helpful. Having it ready encourages us to take our medication and allows them to easily check and remind us if we forget.

- **Simply be there, listen, and keep an open mind.** Sometimes all we need is validation and someone to listen and stay by our side, even if they don't have any advice. Don't be afraid to share exactly what you need from them. Remember, they aren't mind readers.

Informational / Help Books

- Rock Steady: Brilliant Advice from My Bipolar Life by Ellen Forney, Cartoonist
- Take Charge of Bipolar Disorder: A 4-Step Plan for You and Your Loved Ones to Manage the Illness and Create Lasting Stability by Julie A. Fast
- Loving Someone with Bipolar Disorder: Understanding and Helping Your Partner by Julie A. Fast and John D. Preston
- Understanding Bipolar Disorder: The Essential Family Guide by Aimee Daramus, PsyD

Memoirs

- An Unquiet Mind: A Memoir of Moods and Madness by Kay Redfield Jamison
- Mad Like Me: Travels in Bipolar Country by Merryl Hammond, PhD
- Manic: A Memoir by Terri Cheney
- Marbles: Mania, Depression, Michelangelo, and Me: A Graphic Memoir by Ellen Forney, Cartoonist

Podcasts

- Bi-Polar Girl
- Mindful Bipolar
- A Bipolar, A Schizophrenic, and a Podcast
- Bipolar Now
- This is Bipolar
- Let's Talk Bipolar
- Snap Out of It! – The Mental Illness in the Workplace Podcast with Natasha Tracy

Websites

- Beautiful Purpose: A Bipolar Community Group and Nonprofit Organization

  - Join the private group at:
    www.facebook.com/groups/BeautifulPurpose.BP

- DBSA (Depression and Bipolar Support Alliance)

  - https://www.dbsalliance.org

- NAMI (National Alliance on Mental Illness)

  - www.nami.org

- NIMH (National Institute of Mental Health)

  - www.nimh.nih.gov

- bpHope

  - www.bphope.com

  - Subscribe to the their magazine on the website

  - Also available to follow on Facebook

- Mental Health on They Mighty

  - www.themighty.com/topic/mental-health

  - Also available to follow on Facebook

- Bipolar Disorder on The Mighty

  - www.themighty.com/topic/bipolar-disorder

  - Also available to follow on Facebook

- IBF (International Bipolar Foundation)

  - www.ibpf.org

- Suicide & Crisis Lifeline

  - 988Lifeline.org

Famous People with Bipolar Disorder

Dimitri Mihalas (Astrophysicist)

Buzz Aldrin (Second man to walk on the moon)

Isaac Newton (Inventor of Calculus)

Ted Turner (Founder of CNN)

Thomas Eagleton (Lawyer, former United States Senator from Missouri)

Karen McCarthy (Former member of the United States House of Representatives)

John Curtin (14th Prime Minister of Australia)

Linda Hamilton (Sarah Connor of the *Terminator* movies)

Pete Wentz (Musician for *Fall Out Boy*)

Brian Douglas Wilson (Co-founder of *The Beach Boys*)

Bebe Rexha (Singer and songwriter)

Lily Allen (Singer, songwriter, actress, and author)

Stephen Fry (Actor, broadcaster, comedian, director, and writer)

Paul Boyd (Animator who was part of the team that made *Ed, Edd, n Eddy*)

Dusty Springfield (Singer)

Mary Lambert (Singer and songwriter)

Ernest Hemingway (Novelist and journalist)

Catherine Zeta-Jones (Actress)

Demi Lovato (Singer)

Frank Sinatra (Singer and actor)

Russell Brand (Comedian, actor, and author)

Mel Gibson (Actor, director, producer, and screenwriter)

Kanye West (Rapper, record producer, and fashion designer)

Charlie Sheen (Actor)

Mariah Carey (Singer, songwriter, actress, and record producer)

Halsey (Singer)

Robert Downey Jr (Actor and producer)

Krizz Kaliko (Rapper, singer, and songwriter)

Amy Winehouse (Singer and songwriter)

Sia (Singer and songwriter)

Patty Duke (Actress)

Gustav Mahler (Composer)

Wolfgang Mozart (Composer)

Robert Schumann (Composer, pianist, and music critic)

Lord Byron (Poet)

Sylvia Plath (Poet and novelist)

Virginia Woolf (Author)

Edgar Allan Poe (Writer and poet)

Zelda Fitzgerald (Socialite, novelist, painter, and former wife of F. Scott Fitzgerald, a novelist, essayist, and screenwriter)

Aaron Carter (Singer, songwriter, actor, and record producer)

Vincent Van Gogh (Artist)

Tyler Baltierra (Television personality known for being on MTV's *Teen Mom*)

Carrie Fisher (Actress and author)

Ben Stiller (Actor, comedian, producer, director, and writer)

Ben Moody (Musician from *Evanescence)*

G.F. Handel (Composer)

Jelly Roll (Singer and songwriter)

Chyler Leigh (Actress known for her role as Lexie in *Grey's Anatomy*)

Kurt Cobain (Singer and songwriter)

Dolores O'Riordan (Leader of *The Cranberries*)

Steven Page (Former singer for *Barenaked Ladies*)

Justin Furstenfeld (Lead singer of *Blue October*)

Scott Stapp (Former *Creed* frontman)

Michael Angelakos (Former frontman of *Passion Pit*)

David Harbour (Jim Hopper in *Stranger Things)*

Selena Gomez (Singer, actress, producer, and entrepreneur)

Maria Bamford (Actress and comedian)

Margaret Trudeau (Author, actress, former talk show host, and former wife of Pierre Trudeau, the 15th prime minister of Canada)

Everson Griffen (Former NFL player)

Maurice Bernard (Actor, known for his role as Sonny on *General Hospital*)

Jane Pauley (Host for *Today, Dateline*, and *CBS Sunday Morning*)

Maria Bello (Actress, known for her role as Lil Lovelle in *Coyote Ugly*)

Special Thanks To:

Wendi Kelly

ShayAne Hakala

Eric Russell

Andi Sirois

Zoë Pat

Lesley Chapa

Sara Marshall

Taylor Zakrzewski

Gavin Murphy

Rae Dee-ancyger

Ashley Clemente

Francesca Allyn Guy

Taressa McBride

Katie Suzanne Horn

Hakeem Davis

Jerry Post

Brittany Ross

Nadia Massana

Karissa Speroski

Laura Miller

Julia Sayne

Tonya Johnson

Analyn Mattero

Tom Stone

Sooz Golden

Misty Dawn Forest

Lauren Roetman

Robin Schultz

Jessica Ball

Lynn Rose

William Thompson

Jasmin Thomas

Rachel Mandel

Tina Mullins

Laura Ashley

Laura Motyl

Kat Vera

Sasha Winters

Rachel Sessions

Paul Prestigiacomo

Aja Lane

Jess Smith

Sarah Price

Angela Sekelsky

Amber Nightengale

Brittany Krause

Laura Bean

Kenton Hall

Jaime Eldredge

Jennifer Marie Libertini

Pamela Dennis Petteway

Donnetta Sharee Trammel

Pamela Dennis Petteway

Randi Burkett Jeannette

Stacy Patterson Worobey

Susana Itzel Peña Velázquez

Beautiful Purpose: A Bipolar Community

Printed in Great Britain
by Amazon